Health and Fitness for Seniors

Second Edition

W. Newlin Hewson, Ph.D.

Cover Design by Christopher Darden

ISBN: 1515192016
ISBN-13: 978-1515192015

DEDICATION

To my family and colleagues.

CONTENTS

W. Newlin Hewson, Ph.D

ACKNOWLEDGMENTS

I would like to gratefully acknowledge those who have helped and inspired me in compiling this guide:

Travis Combest, Exercise Physiologist

Beth Schultenover, Fitness Instructor

Carol Campbell, Director, Resident Services of Army Distaff Foundation, which operates Knollwood

Kathy Byus, Program Coordinator, Resident Services of Army Distaff Foundation

Claudia Naranjo, Director of Rehabilitation

Nancy Grayson, Registered Dietician

Kristin Natale, Occupational Therapist

Barbara Jolly, Professional Organizer

Elizabeth Compton, Elizabeth "Libby" Janifer, Joan Kane, Lt. Cmdr. William Monagan, Betty Nibley, and Gail Robinson.

Melanie S. Hatter, Editor

"Live fully, a life worth living."

~ W. Newlin Hewson, Ph.D.

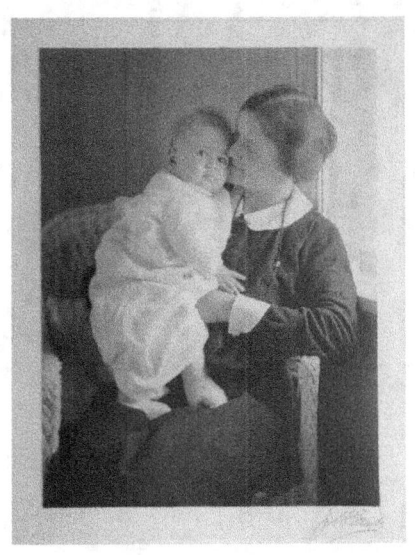

INTRODUCTION

I was born on September 5, 1922, at Pocono Manor Lodge in Pennsylvania, to Dr. and Mrs. William Hewson of Philadelphia. I had an older brother who died in infancy, and four siblings who came after me. I was named William Newlin Hewson, after both my father and maternal grandfather (my friends and family call me Newlie). My late younger brother, Tom, was a retired

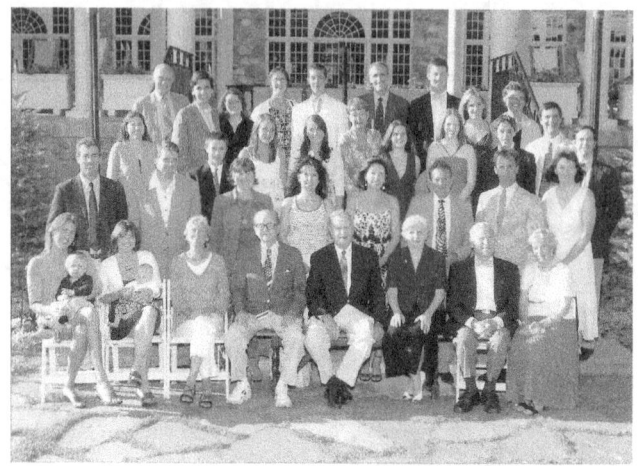

engineer and lived in Florida; my brother Jim is a semi-retired surgeon who lives in Massachusetts; my deceased brother, David, was an environmental specialist; and my only sister, Nancy Jane, is a registered nurse who, early on, rode horse-back to her patients when she lived in Kentucky. She now lives in New Hampshire.

I received my early education at Friends Central School and the Merion Public School. I graduated from the South Kent Boarding School in Connecticut with the class of 1941. As a boy, I became fascinated with sports and airplanes. I was 12 when I began designing and building model planes for endurance competitions.

Through this activity, I developed a healthy respect for mathematics, especially in the double-elliptical wing design. (Mathematics would play a significant role in my career path.) In designing model airplanes, I was especially interested in rubber-band powered stick models that stayed in flight for as long as 30 minutes. With skill and patience, I would design and build stick and fuselage models from scratch, carving a propeller from balsa wood, bending and gluing together tiny pieces to form wing structures, and then carefully applying a covering of microfilm that had 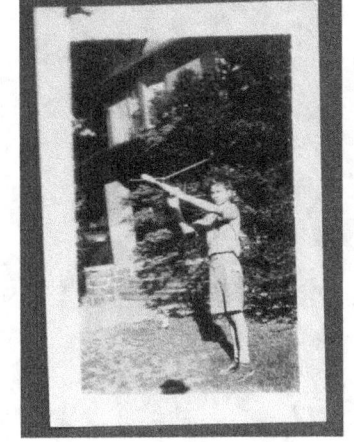 been formed on the still surface of warm water in a bath tub. The results were interesting. At the time, this hobby was very popular, and there were many local and national competitive endurance meets throughout the country for my age group.

The Philadelphia Model Airplane

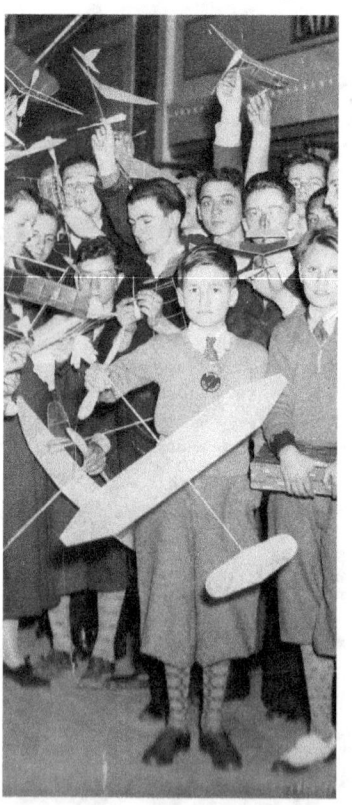 Association was an active organization sponsoring many contests. Classes of competition were divided by age group, surface area of wing, and fuselage type. The ultimate test of the model builder's skill was duration of flight.

I'm proud to say I won or placed in most of these contests. When I was 14, Dad took me to Chicago to participate in the National Champion-ships where I won 4th place with a model that flew for 14 minutes. That same year, I set a National Junior record of 7 minutes and 25 seconds for a class-A stick hydroplane at Atlantic City Convention Hall.

My interest in these types of planes continued for many years, and I developed a healthy respect for the mathematics involved, especially in the double elliptical wing design.

Following high school, I worked briefly with Bendix Aviation before volunteering for the United States Army Air Force and serving in World War II. When discharged in 1946, I entered Gettysburg College, graduating in 1949 with an honors degree in mathematics, and in 1951 graduated as an aerospace officer from the U.S. Air Force's Air University. From there, I joined the Civil Service and first served as an aerospace mathematician at the Naval Air Engineering Center in Philadelphia. I also was an adjunct assistant professor of aerospace, lecturing at St. Joseph's University in Philadelphia.

Some of my early work included a statistical analysis for the certification tests for the world's largest steam catapult aboard the aircraft carrier USS Hancock, and I introduced the statistical discriminate analysis for the design of the definitive mathematics model landing simulation to replace the landing arresting cables on aircraft carrier decks. I later served as a statistical mathematician at the Johnsville Naval Air Development Center, where navigation systems and aircraft costing models were designed. Also, secret Vietnam War statistical analysis was designed there, and I served as a spokesman for the AIRCAB (Flying Ejection Seat) Project. This was a prototype to bring the shot-down pilots

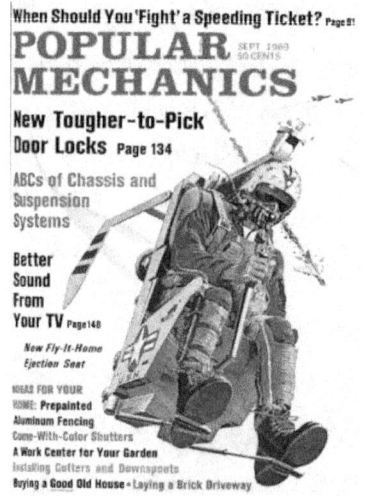

When Should You 'Fight' a Speeding Ticket? Page 91

POPULAR MECHANICS SEPT 1963 50 CENTS

New Tougher-to-Pick Door Locks Page 134

ABCs of Chassis and Suspension Systems

Better Sound From Your TV Page 148

New Fly-It-Home Ejection Seat

IDEAS FOR YOUR HOME: Prepainted Aluminum Fencing Come-With-Color Shutters A Work Center for Your Garden Installing Gutters and Downspouts Buying a Good Old House • Laying a Brick Driveway back to friendly territory by ejecting the pilot's cabin capsule, firing up a mini-jet engine under the pilot's seat and sprouting rotator blades or wings. This project was featured on the cover of *Popular Science* magazine in the fall of 1969.

In 1970, I moved to Washington, D.C., to take a job as a mathematical-statistician with HUD, the federal agency for Housing and Urban Development. While working there, I continued to advance my education through correspondence courses at the Air University and Walden University, then based in Naples, Florida. While at HUD, I did housing research and risk assessment, which led to my doctoral work in a discriminate analysis entitled, "The Prediction of FHA Home Mortgage Foreclosures," resulting in a Ph.D. from Walden University in 1973.

In addition to airplanes, I was also interested in sports, and throughout my life, I have been a strong advocate of fitness, practicing what I preach. I grew up on the tennis courts where my father was a tennis player. He introduced me and my siblings to the sport, and we competed in junior tournaments.

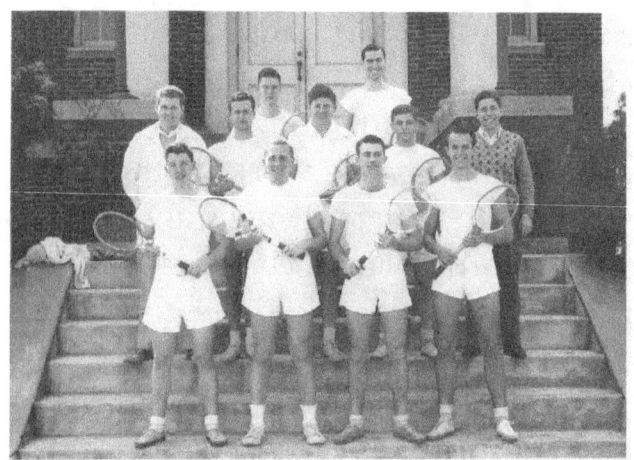

During my high-school years, I played tennis and football and later, after 1970, I joined the Potomac Valley track club. After high school, I began running and race-walking.

Fitness has played an integral role throughout my life.

After retirement, when I moved to

Washington, I devoted my athletic efforts to running, race-walking, and yoga. I sought competition in these pursuits wherever I could find it, and supported the Senior Olympic athletic contests by faithful participation – I competed locally, nationally and internationally for about 17 years, well into my mid-70s.

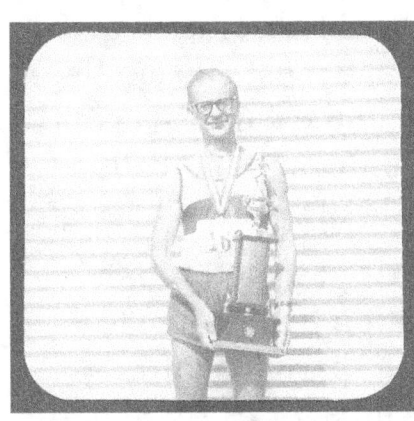

I won eight master's national championship gold medals – seven in running and one in race-walking; set 10 master's national age records (I have received more than 200 master's first-place awards for my age group in local and national competitions). My favorite distance was the 3K in Washington, D.C. at the tidal basin. I competed in many inter-agency competitions, and was especially proud to represent the

United States in the master's World Games in San Diego. I served as captain of six master's national championship running teams and captained the Philadelphia Naval Base tennis team. I am very proud of my athletic ventures and continued to serve as a community health and fitness lecturer until 2001.

We had an athletic family. All of us were tennis players. My brother Jim, the surgeon, was also the most outstanding all-around athlete in the family – he did well in tennis, running and football during his high-school years.

For inspiration, I gathered some statistical information that led me to predict that my life span – barring unforeseeable circumstances – will be 107 years! Whether that will happen or not, there is an opportunity to expand our life spans beyond 100, if we pursue aerobic (heart-lung) activities for a healthier, longer life.

My interest in the aging process resulted in my receiving Board

Certification as a gerontology lecturer in 2001 from the University of the District of Columbia. As I get older, I see so many who are advancing in age who are not faring as well as they might. Too many are allowing themselves to wither away.

As a resident at the Knollwood Military Officers Retirement Residence in Washington, D.C., I want to share my health insights, fitness knowledge, and experience with this community and those beyond to help everyone live a healthier, longer life.

It's never too late to get started on a healthier life path. This book will give you some guidance on how to create a more enjoyable, productive and active lifestyle, no matter what your age.

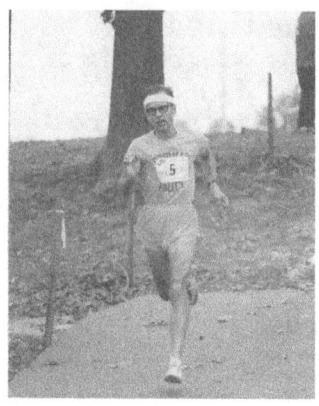

REASONS TO EXERCISE

"A sedentary life is not a good lifestyle for longevity. You have to be mentally and physically active. Too many people are not contributing positively with their lifestyle; instead they could be making more friends and concentrating on things that will benefit everybody. Too many people are not living – they're simply existing and not making positive contributions. They've got to live better and healthier lives."

~ W. Newlin Hewson, Ph.D.

Physical Benefits:

- Improved efficiency of heart and lungs
- Improved muscle tone
- Improved agility and coordination
- Improved resistance to muscular injury (especially lower back pain)
- More energy for both work and recreation
- Decreased body fat
- Increased strength
- Increased stamina
- Improved posture
- Greater flexibility
- Reduced resting heart rate
- Reduced resting blood pressure decrease cholesterol levels
- Reduced recovery time after exercise delays the process of aging
- Reduced risk of heart disease
- Increased oxygen consumption (aerobic capacity)

- Maintain ideal weight
- Ability to perform daily chores of living without undue fatigue or strain

Psychological Benefits:

- Reduced tension and stress
- Improved ability for a sounder sleep
- Improved self-image and self confidence
- Reduced depression and anxiety
- Increased positive outlook on life
- Concentrate better and think more creatively
- Overall feeling of well-being

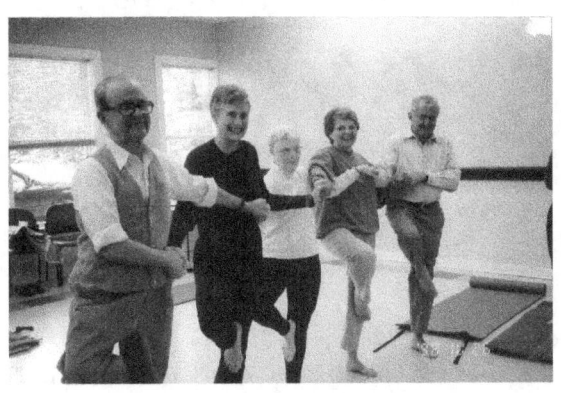

GETTING STARTED – YOU'RE NEVER TOO OLD

"Ask yourself, what have you done today to get more out of life and raise the spirits of others to make a better world for all of us? Are you encouraging others to contribute? Society needs positive contributions – all who can contribute, should. There's an awful lot you can do for yourself. You just have to get out there and enjoy the world around you."

~ W. Newlin Hewson, Ph.D.

One of the best things you can do for yourself is join a walking group. I see

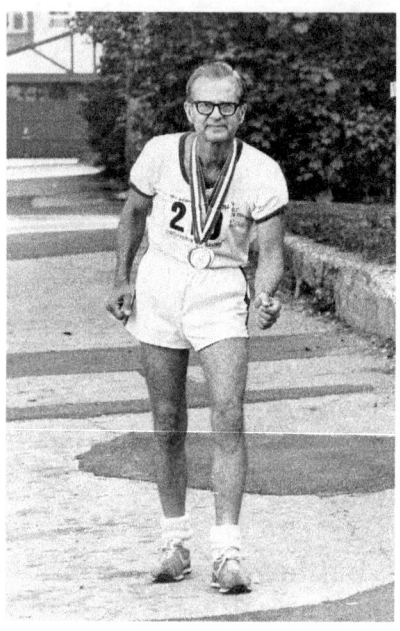

walkers out each Saturday morning, enjoying the nature around them. In this area, you can see deer and Canada geese all around us. It's good for adults and youngsters being able to watch the animals come and go and the birds flying overhead. It's a wonderful thing to simply watch the clouds and see the assortment of shapes they make. It's so important to enjoy the sunshine and get a good dose of Vitamin D. You do have to be careful when you go out into the sun. The most damaging hours are between 11 a.m. and 3 p.m. I usually go out after 3 p.m.

Too many elderly people stay inside or, worse, in bed. I encourage anyone I see who isn't taking advantage of this great world around us. Although I can no longer drive – at my age I've lost my privilege to renew my driver's license – I take advantage of the buses provided here at Knollwood to get out and go to events. Many assisted living facilities offer a great many ways for the residents to stay active, including exercise equipment, massage therapy and fitness classes.

For those not in a senior home environment, there are many opportunities in your community available free or at a reduced rate for seniors. Visit your local library, which is a great resource for what's going on around you.

To keep in shape, I use the exercycle while I'm watching TV. People need more vigorous exercise than just

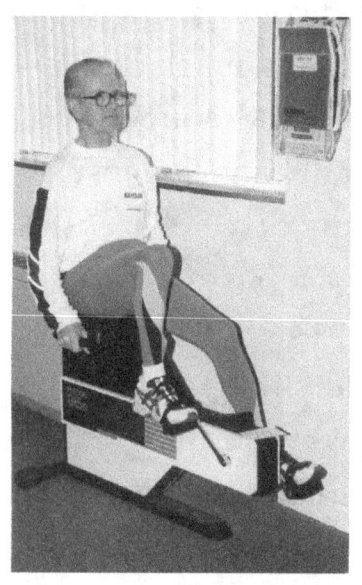

strolling or slow walking. Unfortunately, many are not getting the exercise they need to strengthen and maintain their bodies. Too many people are passing on who are not taking advantage of these things. I know one gentleman who is using the assisted living facility like a hospice. He is two years older than I am, he's getting thin and frail and getting cranky and difficult to deal with – exercising would give him a more positive outlook.

When looking at how to get started, avoid dangerous forms of physical activity, for example, contact sports because players are getting too intense. Aerobic exercise that reaches a pulse of 125 is appropriate for septuagenarians. Chair exercises, pool therapy or pool aerobics are excellent forms of exercise.

Here are some simple exercises you can do while watching TV.

Muscle Conditioning Exercises
– In or With a Chair

When first beginning this chair exercise routine, start with one set (group) of 10 reps (times) and then progress in the next two to four weeks to 2-3 sets of 10 reps, if you feel okay. For progression, usually in 2-4 weeks if the exercise program becomes easier, maintain three sets then increase to between 12-15 reps. If this becomes easier, add an ankle weight, starting with 1 lb.

Make sure to have a day of rest in between your exercise conditioning days to allow the muscles to recover. For example, your routine could be on Monday, Wednesday and Friday. The minimum amount of days you want to perform exercise conditioning is two days a week, but aim for three days a week.

Keep in mind that you can perform aerobic conditioning, such as walking, on almost all days of the week if you feel comfortable and can be included on the same day as your muscle conditioning program. Make sure to consult your physician before starting an exercise program, and make sure to increase gradually with your exercise.

Knee Raise

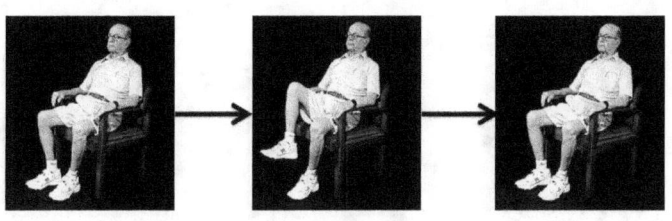

10 Repetitions

Leg Extension

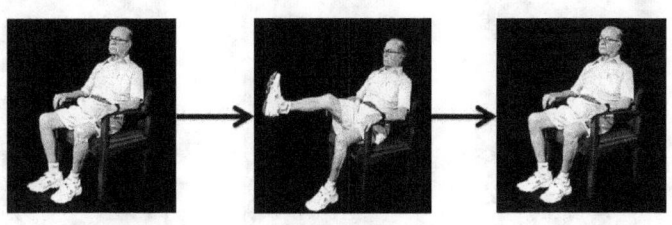

10 Repetitions

Toe Raise

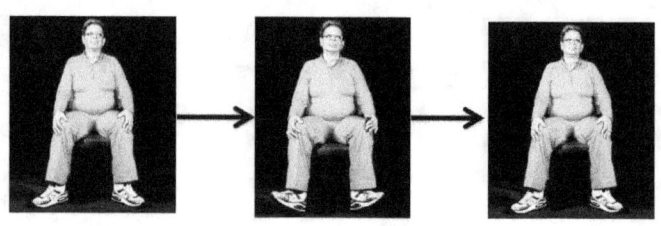

10 Repetitions

Hip Flex

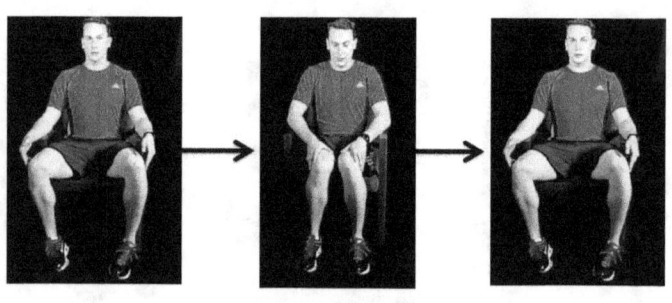

10 Repetitions

Leg Curl

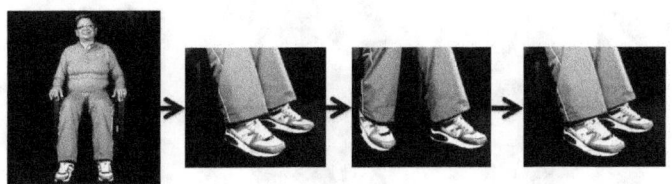

10 Repetitions

Calf Raise

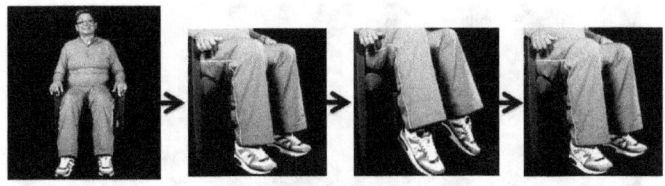

10 Repetitions

Sit to Stand

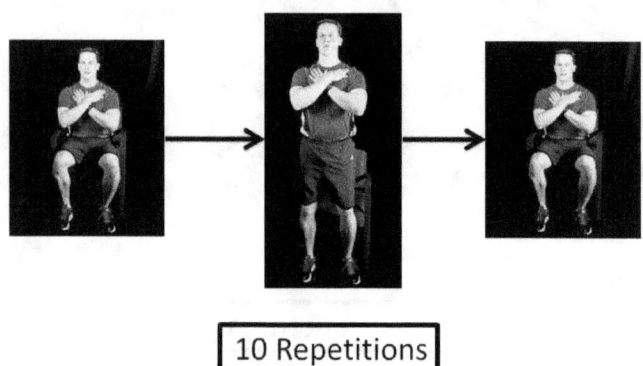

10 Repetitions

Balance Exercise

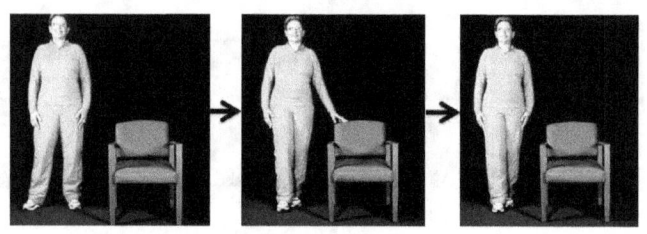

10 Repetitions

Here are some pictures taken from our Chair Pilates class at Knollwood:

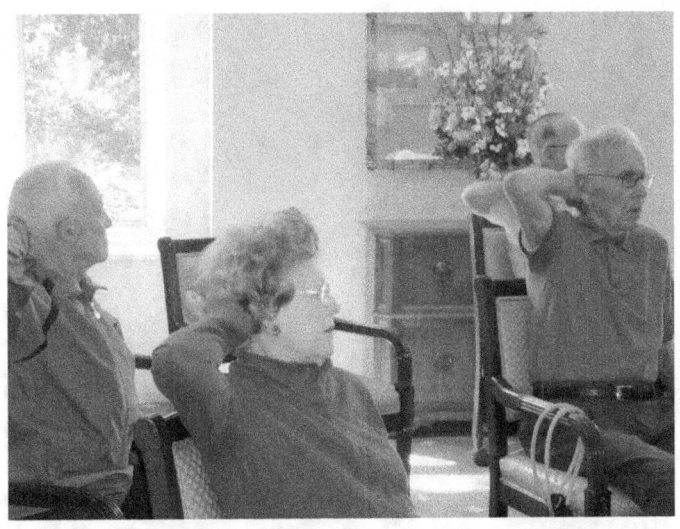

This is a neck stretch that we do in the beginning of our program, and can be performed with or without using the arm. Place one hand behind the head and open the elbow as wide as possible. While exhaling, slowly turn the head in the opposite direction. Hold for a full breath in and out, then on the second breath while exhaling, open the arm a bit wider and turn the head deeper in to the stretch. Inhale, then exhale as you slowly close the elbow and return the head to starting position. Repeat on the other side.

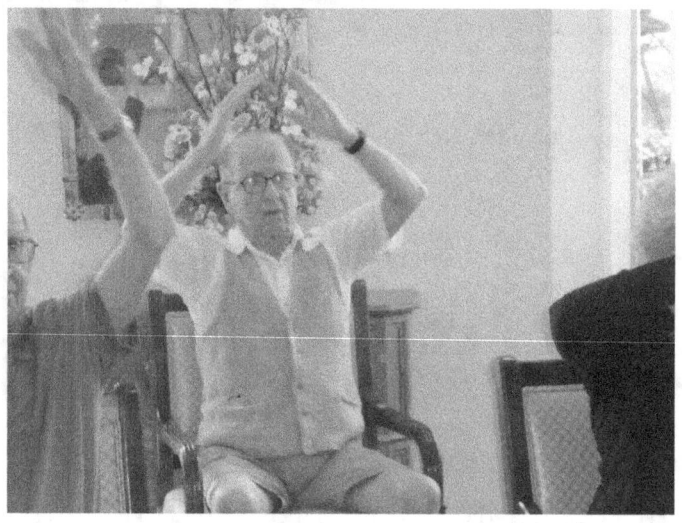

To work on range of motion for the arms, start with your arms next to the chair and raise them over your head while exhaling; inhale as the arms are lowered. Repeat 4-5 times.

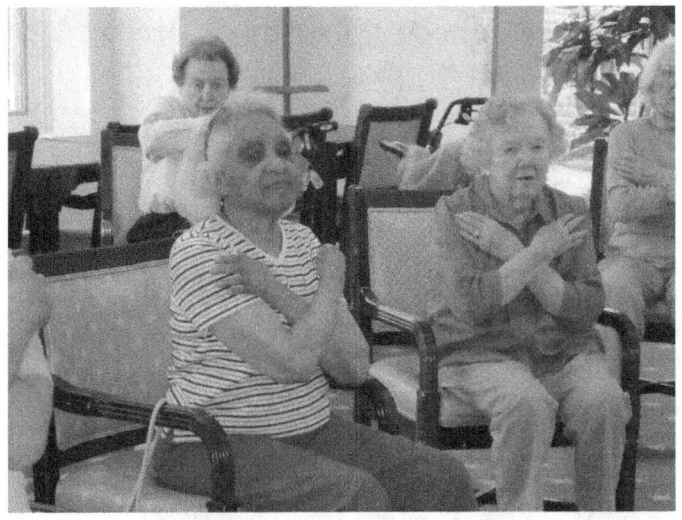

For a modified sit-up: While sitting on the edge of the chair, with your feet firmly planted on the floor and knees at a 90-degree angle, cross your arms at the chest and bring your pelvis upward while also bringing the belly in toward your spine. Your lower back will naturally curve. While inhaling slowly lean back to touch the back of your chair. Exhale as you straighten the spine and come forward to the starting position. If it is too difficult to get back to the starting position, adjust by sitting farther back in the chair. It is important that your feet remain planted on the

floor throughout the entire exercise.
Repeat 8 -10 times.

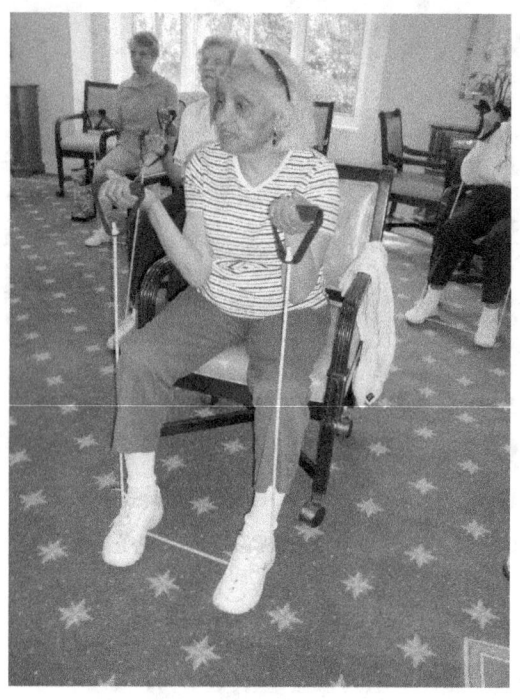

To work the biceps using resistance
bands, sit with feet hip distance apart,
place the band firmly under the arch of
both feet and hold the end of the bands
with palms facing upward. Elbows are
tight at the side and the forearms are
lifted in a slow and controlled manner.

Exhale as you lift and inhale as you lower. Repeat 10-12 times. To increase resistance, widen the feet beyond hip distance. Only go as far as is comfortable.

For a comprehensive resource on Exercise & Physical Activity, the National Institute on Aging provides a complementary guide that's available by visiting NIH's website at www.NIHSeniorHealth.gov or by calling 1 (800) 222-2225.

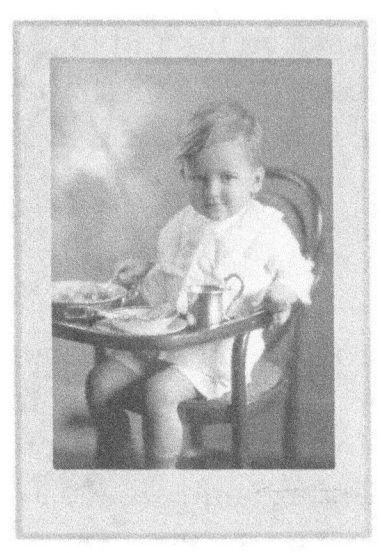

DON'T FORGET ABOUT DIET

"People are getting chubbier. I see so many with excessive waistlines. We must be more thoughtful about what we eat. There's too much starchy stuff that we put into our bodies. People are just not thinking. They're thinking about their past and not about creating a better future and how to contribute in a way that makes life more enjoyable for everyone."

~ W. Newlin Hewson, Ph.D.

Generally as we age, our metabolism slows somewhat, but we should continue to ensure we are eating properly. The Jean Mayer USDA Human Nutrition Research Center on Aging (USDA HNRCA) at Tufts University created MyPlate for Older Adults, which corresponds with the 2010 Dietary Guidelines for Americans. These dietary guidelines were released by the federal government to promote health, reduce the risk of chronic diseases, and reduce the prevalence of overweight and obesity through improved nutrition and physical activity. The guidelines focus on balancing calories with physical activity.

According to Alice H. Lichtenstein, senior scientist and director of the Cardiovascular Nutrition Laboratory at the USDA HNRCA, MyPlate for Older Adults offers examples of foods high in vitamins and minerals per serving and is intended to be a guide for healthy, older adults living independently and looking for examples of good food choices and physical activities.

Here are foods, fluids and physical activities represented on My Plate for Older Adults:

- Bright-colored vegetables such as carrots and broccoli.

- Deep-colored fruit such as berries and peaches.

- Whole, enriched and fortified grains and cereals such as brown rice and 100% whole wheat bread.

- Low- and non-fat dairy products such as yogurt and low-lactose milk.

- Dry beans and nuts, fish, poultry, lean meat and eggs.

- Liquid vegetable oils, soft spreads low in saturated and *trans* fat, and spices to replace salt.

- Fluids such as water and fat-free milk.

- Physical activity such as walking, resistance training and light cleaning.

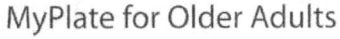

MyPlate for Older Adults

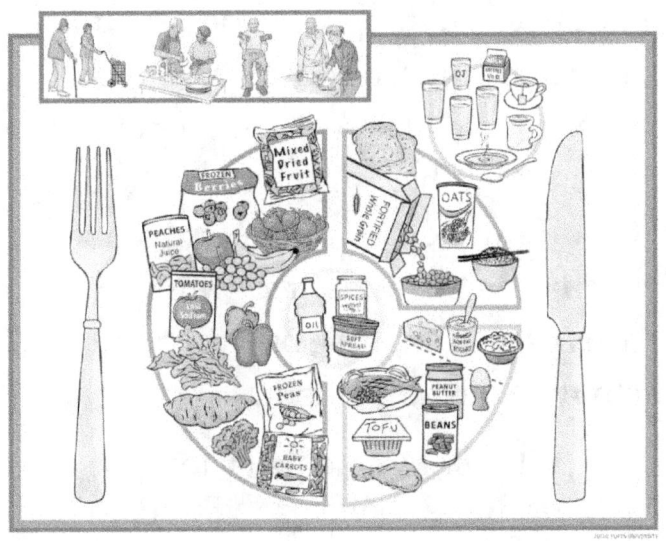

MyPlate for Older Adults suggests eating whole, enriched and fortified grains because they are high in fiber; plant-based protein options such as beans and tofu as well as fish and lean meat; and vegetable oils and soft spreads as alternatives to foods high in animal fats, which are higher in saturated and *trans* fat.

Supplementing Your Diet

Although most of us cannot get the amount of vitamins our body requires naturally, you can consider supplements. These do not replace foods but, rather, supplement the diet. Fish oil supplements have proven effective as they stabilize brainwave patterns and increase overall brain activity. Here are others:

- Vitamin A – helps vision and promotes bone growth, tooth development, and helps maintain healthy skin, hair, and mucous membranes.

- Vitamin B1 – helps body cells convert carbohydrates into energy; essential for the functioning of the heart, muscles, and nervous system.

- Vitamin B3 – assists in the functioning of the digestive system, skin and nerves; important for the conversion of food to energy.

- Vitamin B6 – plays a role in the creation of antibodies in the immune system; helps maintain normal nerve function and helps form red blood cells.

- Vitamin B12 – important for metabolism; helps with the formation of red blood cells and in the maintenance of the central nervous system.

- Vitamin C – plays a significant role as an antioxidant, protecting body tissue from the damage of oxidation; is an effective antiviral agent.

- Vitamin D – promotes absorption of calcium and magnesium, which are essential for the normal development of healthy teeth and bones.

- Vitamin E – plays a significant role as an antioxidant, protecting body tissue from the damage of oxidation; important in forming red blood cells and the use of vitamin K.

- Folic Acid – helps produce red blood cells and tissue cells; helps promote normal growth and a healthy intestinal tract.

- Magnesium – needed for bone, protein, making new cells, activating B vitamins, relaxing nerves and muscles, clotting blood, and in energy production.

- Selenium – part of several enzymes necessary for the body to properly function; acts as an antioxidant that works in conjunction with vitamin E.

- Zinc – important for protein and carbohydrate metabolism, immune system, wound healing, growth and vision.

In his book, *Healthy Aging – A lifelong Guide to Your Physical and Spiritual Well-Being*, Andrew Weil, M.D., recommends what he calls the "Anti-inflammatory Diet." He says this is less a diet plan and more a way of eating as part of a healthy lifestyle – eating foods that discourage unnecessary inflammation within the body that can cause disease. He offers a convincing argument for paying closer attention to the food we put into our bodies.

Dr. Weil says to eat less meat, poultry and foods of animal origin. Eat more vegetable protein, such as soy, beans and lentils, whole grains, seeds, and nuts. And he suggests that if you eat fish, to avoid varieties that may carry high toxic contaminants such as mercury and polychlorinated biphenyls (PCBs). Reduce saturated fat by eating less butter, cream, cheese and other full-fat dairy products, unskinned chicken, fatty meats, and products made with coconut and palm kernel oils. Reduce foods made with wheat flour and sugar, especially bread and snacks including chips and pretzels.

In general, Dr. Weil encourages you to:

- Aim for variety
- Include as much fresh food as possible.
- Minimize your consumption of processed foods and fast food.
- Eat an abundance of fruits and vegetables.

Overall, his book provides excellent advice for living well as we get older. It's worth a read.

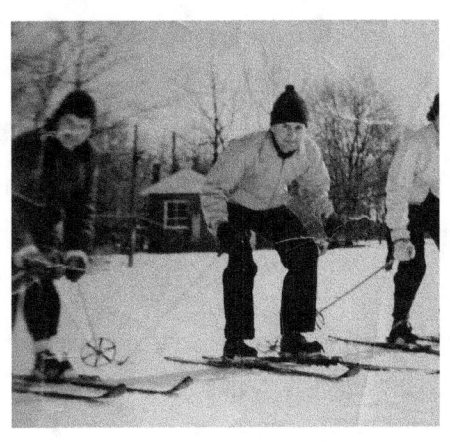

WORKING OUT THE INSIDE

"Too many people walk looking downcast. The emphasis should be on looking up and out. Get involved and enjoy a social experience, such as dancing or going to a performance or community activity. Do things with your hands, for example, join a crafts club. Get a routine established and enjoy the environment. Find ways to look positively at what you're doing; be with people who are enjoying activities with others and engage with the world around you, enlightening and stimulating others to enjoy life as it should be lived."

~ W. Newlin Hewson, Ph.D.

While you work on your outer body, don't neglect to work on your inner body, too – maintaining a healthy state of mind is just as important as keeping your body in good shape. In this chapter, we take a look at how to de-stress your life, keep depression at bay, and fight memory loss.

Type A personalities are often described as being competitive and workaholics, but while this drive for success can be good for business, it can be detrimental to your health. In the late 1950s, cardiologists Meyer Friedman and R.H. Rosenman developed the theory that Type A personalities may be connected to coronary heart disease.

In his 1996 book, *Type A Behavior: Its Diagnosis and Treatment,* Dr. Friedman notes two major symptoms associated with Type A behavior:

- free-floating hostility
- time urgency and impatience

While Type A behavior is alarmingly prevalent, its negative effects can be counteracted. First, let's consider who would benefit from treatment. There are several groups:

Group I

- Survivors of one or more heart attacks
- Those suffering from heartbeat irregularities
- Angina pectoris sufferers (blocked arteries)
- Those with coronary symptoms but whose treadmill tests are positive

Group II – Those suffering maturity onset diabetes

Group III – Triple risk people

- Smokers

- Hypersensitive
- High blood cholesterol

Group IV – Hypertensive or people with positive history of coronary heart disease.

Group V – Those outwardly expressing aggravation, irritation, anger, and impatience. The first four groups of Type A behavior are <u>acutely</u> in need of behavior modification to prevent heart attacks, but this last group is <u>seriously</u> in need of behavior modification.

How to Shift from Type A to Type B

Dr. Friedman suggested that Type A personalities should take things a bit slower to counteract the effects of stress on their bodies and minds, and work toward a healthier perspective. Here are some ideas to consider if you are a Type A personality, or if you know someone who is:

- Each morning remind yourself of all projects that don't need time deadlines.
- Before beginning a task ask yourself if the task's execution will matter six years from now. Must it be done right away and can it be delegated?
- Do one thing at a time.
- Drive in the slow lane.
- Walk, talk and eat more slowly.
- For a whole workday, move your whole arms not just the fingers when writing.
- Don't interfere with a person doing his job slower than you would.
- Communicate with a friend of a different profession and try to find a subject of mutual interest.
- Listen to others and gain from them.
- Listen to two people on two separate occasions without interrupting once.

- Before speaking, ask yourself, do I really have something to say; does anyone wish to hear it; is this the right time to say it?
- Ask a family member what they did for the day and listen to their answer.
- After a meal with friends, take note of their concerns and encourage them to talk about their interests.
- Record an hour of dinner table conversation and play it back.
- Find a long supermarket line and get to the end of it – observe and ask yourself questions about others in the queue.
- Use adjectives instead of numbers to express your thoughts and eliminate "how much" and "how many."
- Read novels and avocational-related books.
- Seek beauty in all phases of your life, adding smiles and metaphors

for color and life to your conversations.

- At least weekly, ask yourself: does haste ever aid good judgment and correct decisions?
- Place more emphasis on time rather than on money.
- Review the notes before the next meeting to enhance genuine interest.
- Visit a museum, park, zoo or aquarium.
- Note the components of a tree, flower, sunset or dawn.
- Establish daily life rituals – i.e., repeat pleasant or notable events or activities.
- Devote 15 minutes to planning a new avocation.
- Recall past times and events for 15 minutes.
- Do absolutely nothing but listen to music for 15 minutes.

- At bedtime ask yourself these questions:

- What did I do right today, and
- What is worth remembering?

Don't Let Depression Get You Down

Types of Depression

- Dysthymia – Life's normal rhythmic pattern is affected
- Seasonal Affective Disorder (SAD) – Affects sleep and eating
- Bipolar Disorder – Dramatic mood swings

Fighting Depression – Accentuate the positive

A good night's sleep combats depression

- Stick to a sleep schedule, going to bed at the same time every night and rising at the same time in the morning

- Exercise but not too late in the day.

- Avoid caffeine, nicotine, alcohol, large meals and beverages before bed

- Avoid medicines that delay or disrupt your sleep, if possible.

- Don't take naps after 3 p.m.

- Relax before bedtime, for example, take a hot bath before you head to bed.

- Have a good sleeping environment, for example, no noise or distractions; play soft music, read a book to relax you; before sleeping watch relaxing and enjoyable TV rather than a crime drama.

- Have the right sunlight exposure – spend limited time in the sun, avoiding the hours between 11 a.m. and 3 p.m. when the sun is at its hottest.

- Don't lie in bed awake – if you can't sleep, practice meditation or listen to restful music with an automatic shut off. Also, make sure to empty your bladder before heading to bed so you're not disturbed in the night. Do see a doctor if you continue to have trouble sleeping.

Positive relationships with people and pets

- Positive relationships generate higher levels of oxytocin (the "feel good" hormone), which in turn helps wounds heal faster, increases pain tolerance, lowers stress hormones, and reduces blood pressure.

- Studies have shown that pets increase the survival rate for cardiac patients, decrease stress, reduce bone loss, lower cholesterol levels, and improve blood circulation.

- Think of blessings that have come your way and how to share those blessings; think good thoughts and share with others – there's a lot of positive sharing that can be done.

Get the giggles – Laughter lengthens life

- Boosts immune and circulatory system

- Enhances oxygen intake

- Stimulates the heart and lungs

- Relaxes muscles throughout the body

- Triggers release of endorphins

- Eases digestion/soothes stomach aches

- Relieves pain

- Balances blood pressure

- Improves mental functions

- Improves overall attitude

- Reduces stress/tension

- Promotes relaxation and improves sleep
- Enhances quality of life
- Strengthens social bonds and relationships
- Produces a general sense of well being

Natural and herbal remedies can help stimulate a positive outlook

- St. John's Wort (only with doctor's approval)
- Omega-3 fatty acids
- SAM-e (S-adenosylmethionine)
- Folic Acid
- 5-HTP (5-Hydroxytryptophan)
- Healthy diet
- Exercise, for example, yoga
- Talk therapy – talk to friends and, if needed, make an appointment to see a doctor
- Acupuncture

- Massage
- Meditation (see below)
- Hobbies

How to Manage Stress

Unfortunately, we all experience stress and it doesn't go away as you age.

For some, simply getting older may cause stress due to declining health, losing friends and family members, adjusting to retirement and possibly a decreased income, and being alone. As we age, we may experience a loss of control over our lives, reduced physical strength and coordination, and lose our sense of purpose in life.

Short-term stress causes the body to respond with increased heartbeat, breathing and muscle tension. This is the "fight or flight" response to what the body perceives as a threat. Stress causes your body to release stress hormones, which stimulate your brain and body. Over a long time, that type of stimulation can be dangerous.

Long term stress increases your risk for heart disease, high blood pressure, stroke, digestive problems and sleep disorders. Many seniors are already at a greater risk for these conditions and too much stress may be too much to handle. Studies show that long-term stress can damage brain cells, leading to depression.

Symptoms of stress may include anxiety, sadness, trouble eating and sleeping, aches and pains, and weight loss.

Many of the techniques to fight depression can be used to combat stress. One method in particular that I would like to highlight here is meditation.

Meditation Can Benefit You

In the 1970s, Dr. Herbert Benson, founder of the Benson-Henry Institute for Mind Body Medicine at Massachusetts General Hospital, found that meditation reduced metabolism, rate of breathing, heart rate and brain activity. In his book, *The Relaxation Response*, Dr. Benson describes the scientific benefits of relaxation, noting that regular practice can be an effective treatment for many stress-related disorders.

A five-year study is underway by John Denninger, a psychiatrist at Harvard Medical School, on how meditation and yoga affect genes and brain activity in the chronically stressed. The study, which started in 2013, is using neuro-imaging and genomics technology to measure physiological changes in greater detail. Denninger, who also directs research at the Benson-Henry Institute for Mind Body Medicine, says that meditation has a biological effect throughout the body and not just in the brain. But we don't need to wait for his results to incorporate this practice into our own lives.

Types of Meditation

There are many ways to reach a relaxed state of being. Here are a few different forms of meditation:

Guided meditation uses imagery or visualization, where you form mental images of places or situations you find relaxing. You use as many senses as possible, such as smells, sights, sounds and textures. This method is often led by a guide or teacher in person or on a recording.

Mantra meditation is where you silently repeat a calming word, thought or phrase to prevent distracting thoughts.

Transcendental meditation is similar to mantra meditation in that you repeat a word, sound or phrase. The goal is to allow your body to settle into a state of deep rest and relaxation.

Mindfulness meditation is based on being aware of the present moment and accepting each moment as it comes. Focus on what you experience during meditation, such as the flow of your breath. Observe your thoughts and emotions, but let them pass without judgment.

Let's Get Started

Meditation means turning your attention away from distracting thoughts, calming the mind and developing inner peace.

If you are new to meditation, a great place to start is by simply focusing on your breath. Find a quiet place and sit in a comfortable position. You can sit in the traditional cross-legged posture, but sitting in a chair is fine, too. The key is to keep your back straight so you don't become sluggish or sleepy. Breathe naturally, preferably through the nose, without attempting to control your breath. Be aware of the sensation of the breath as it enters and leaves your nostrils. You can add a mantra, for example, "so hum," which connects you and your breath with the universe. As you inhale say, silently in your mind: "So," and when you exhale, say: "hum."

In the beginning your mind will be active, but do your best to let the thoughts go. You may get distracted by noise or more thoughts, but keep returning your focus to your breathing and/or the mantra. Don't engage in an inner dialogue with yourself. Sit for as long as you can, even if it's only a few minutes. Aim for five to 10 minutes and as you get more comfortable add a few minutes each session. Over time you'll find yourself sitting for longer periods.

And don't judge yourself harshly if you think you're not "getting it." There really is nothing to get. Simply relax and breathe.

How to Avoid Memory Loss

This is an area we are all concerned about. We get a little nervous when we misplace our keys or forget a phone number we've dialed a hundred times before. Could it be a sign of something wrong? Let's take a look at our natural memory processes and when to get further evaluation. Let's also consider strategies to actively maintain the memories we have.

Here are 10 questions to ask yourself if you feel your memory could be slipping. Each of these areas is a part of the normal process of aging and not necessarily an ominous sign of mental deterioration.

1. Is it difficult for you to remember names of your friends most of the time?

2. Is it hard to recall the day of the week?

3. Does it take a very long time or is it impossible for you to learn something new?

4. Do you repeat yourself often?

5. Do you feel tired all the time?

6. Do you need caffeine or other stimulants to get you started or keep you going?

7. Do little things bother you much more than they used to?

8. Do you frequently miss your appointments?

9. Do you find yourself searching for something and you forget what you are looking for?

10. Is it difficult for you to add numbers without a pen and paper?

The good news is that not all forgetfulness is caused by Alzheimer's disease. Not all memory impairment reaches the severity of dementia. What looks like significant memory loss can be caused by treatable, even reversible, conditions. Significant memory loss is not an inevitable result of aging. The brain is capable of producing new brain pathways at any age, and new learning can occur at any age. To a large extent, maintaining a healthy memory is under your control.

Many brain functions are largely unaffected by normal aging, such as:

- How to do the things you've always done and do often,

- The wisdom and knowledge you've acquired from life experience,

- Your innate common sense,

- The ability to form reasonable arguments and judgments, and

- The ability to learn new skills and make them routine, though it might take longer.

The following types of memory lapses are normal among older adults and generally are not considered warning signs of dementia:

- Forgetting where you left things you use regularly, such as glasses or keys,

- Forgetting names of acquaintances or figures in the news,

- Occasionally forgetting an appointment,

- Having trouble remembering what you just read,

- Walking into a room and forgetting why you entered,

- Forgetting the details of conversations,

- Becoming easily distracted,

- Not quite able to retrieve information you have "on the tip of your tongue," and

- Blocking one memory with a similar one, such as calling a grandson by your son's name.

Mild Cognitive Impairment

When the information you forget is no longer trivial and your forgetfulness begins to have consequences – you miss your doctor's appointment more than once or blank on your home address – your memory loss is beyond that of "normal" memory loss due to aging and may be diagnosed as mild cognitive impairment.

The memory lapses are similar to those of someone in the earliest stage of Alzheimer's and some experts see it as a precursor to Alzheimer's or other form of dementia.

When memory loss becomes so pervasive and severe that it disrupts your work, hobbies, social activities, family relationships, you may be experiencing the warning signs of Alzheimer's disease, another disorder that causes dementia, or a condition that mimics dementia.

Alzheimer's

Alzheimer's disease is the most common type of dementia. It is a progressive and degenerative disease, which means that it gets worse over time.

Currently, it is estimated that as many as 5.4 million people in the U.S. have it. This number is expected to grow over the next 50 years as the population ages and life spans increase.

When someone has Alzheimer's disease, nerve cells die in areas of the brain that are vital to cognition, which may include memory, judgment, thinking and other mental abilities. Connections between nerve cells are disrupted. In addition, there are lower levels of some of the chemicals in the brain that carry messages back and forth between nerve cells. Through research, we are learning more about how Alzheimer's affects the brain. We do not yet know how to prevent or cure it, but we do know how to treat its symptoms.

For more specific information on Alzheimer's disease, visit the Alzheimer's Association website at www.alz.org or call 1 (800) 272-3900.

When to See a Doctor

It's time to consult a doctor when memory lapses become frequent enough or sufficiently noticeable to concern you or a family member. If you get to that point, make an appointment to talk with your doctor and have a thorough physical exam. The doctor will ask you questions about your memory including how long you or others have noticed a problem, what kinds of things have been difficult to remember, did this happen gradually or suddenly, and if you are having trouble doing ordinary things.

Prevent Memory Loss and Fight Brain Aging!

The brain is an incredible organ. It has served us well and will continue to do if we are proactive in taking charge of our health habits. Here are a variety of strategies that keep our memories sharp:

Cardiovascular Exercises

More than anything, getting oxygen to brain cells ensures they can do their job. Getting at least a 20- to 30-minute workout four times a week is minimally beneficial to our health in general. Using the treadmill and the heart monitor can let you know if you are in the target heart rate zone for an adequate workout.

I am always encouraged when I see residents taking advantage of the outdoors by walking, playing tennis or golfing.

Debates

By engaging in a debate, you are challenging your brain's ability to generate a stimulating conversation that requires rapid thinking and high levels of focus. To start one, just ask someone, "who should be president?"

Nutrition

Eating healthy is a huge factor in determining a healthy brain. The food you put in your body is what your brain is forced to work with. There are many foods that have been proven beneficial for memory. Foods that are high in fiber and those high in antioxidants can keep the brain healthy, for example: fish, especially sardines; tomatoes; strawberries; cherries; whole grains; and nuts are good. (See previous chapter for more on nutrition.)

Here are some things to keep in mind for how you can impact your memory diet:

- **Improved Memory Capacity**
  - ✓ Ginkgo Biloba
  - ✓ Ginseng
  - ✓ St. John's Wort
  - ✓ Curries reduce free radicals
  - ✓ Fruit juice increases antioxidants

- **Detrimental to Memory in Excess**
  - ✓ Sugar
  - ✓ Cholesterol
    - ▪ Saturated Fat
    - ▪ Triglycerides
  - ✓ Caffeine

Strategies for Brain Health

- Try doing a crossword puzzle or a jigsaw puzzle. On the fourth floor of my building, a resident set up a jigsaw puzzle for anyone to stop by and put a few pieces in place. Puzzles cause us to think critically and naturally increase brain activity. Playing brain fitness games challenges your brain and promotes quick thinking.

- Reading something challenging every day stimulates synapse growth (electrical and chemical impulses in the brain) and increases thinking ability. Using and challenging your brain helps prevent you from losing it!

- TV promotes less mental activity and a lazy brain. Watch educational programs in moderation. It's okay to be entertained, but when it becomes a crutch and takes away from other activities, turn it off.

- Meditation has been known to reduce stress, lower blood pressure, promote positive thinking, reduce depression and anxiety, and increase memory, alertness, and task-performance. About 20 minutes of meditation – freeing your mind from thoughts and not trying to solve problems – can be as good as a nap and refresh and help you focus.

- Positive thinking is a trait associated with longevity and a healthy brain. Just 10 minutes a day focusing on positive thoughts will make you naturally feel more energized and happy.

- Getting enough sleep is good for the brain, yet we don't do it. At least eight hours is most beneficial for health.

- It's never a good idea to unnecessarily stress yourself out. Some stress is healthy, but too much kills brain cells from excess amounts of cortisol (known as the stress hormone). Use techniques like deep breathing to reduce the effects of stress.

- Writing is a great activity to keep your mind stimulated and reflect on daily activities. Writing definitely stimulates the brain in profound ways that talking does not.

- Get outside and get some sunshine. Exchange smiles with a stranger and experience the beauty of nature. Just being outside can have a significant impact on your mood and brain.

- Neurofeedback – a procedure that stimulates positive brain waves – promotes brainwave flexibility and the conscious control of mental activity to reduce stress and increase focus.

- Listening to music is severely underrated as it stimulates the right hemisphere in the brain, which is associated with emotions and creativity. Play tunes while exercising or writing.

- Playing sports competitively is known to benefit the player's brain.

- Change it up, do something different! Your brain grows new connections when its environment changes. Experience more in life, stop following the same routine. Variety is the spice of life.

- Know your blood pressure; get it checked regularly and avoid salty foods. Lowered blood pressure is associated with a reduced Alzheimer's risk.

- Hang out with true friends. Being with people who truly care for you and always love you benefits you emotionally and mentally.

- Get organized and plan your day. Write effective notes, make a to-do list, use monthly or weekly calendars, get an electronic organizer, or use Post-it notes. By planning at least a couple of activities in advance for each day, you will always have something to look forward to. This is good for your brain because it keeps you excited and wards off depression.

- Live for the moment! Take whatever action you need to do "today" to make your dreams come true "tomorrow."

- Drugs not under doctor's orders are bad for you. Drugs kill brain cells, make you naturally more stressed out, and decrease healthy brain activity.

- Alcohol isn't good for brain function. Either cut alcohol consumption or make a conscious effort to reduce your intake.

Try to remember ...

Look, Snap, and Connect

- **LOOK –** Actively observe what you want to learn
- **SNAP –** Create mental snapshots of memories
- **CONNECT –** Associate two mental snaps

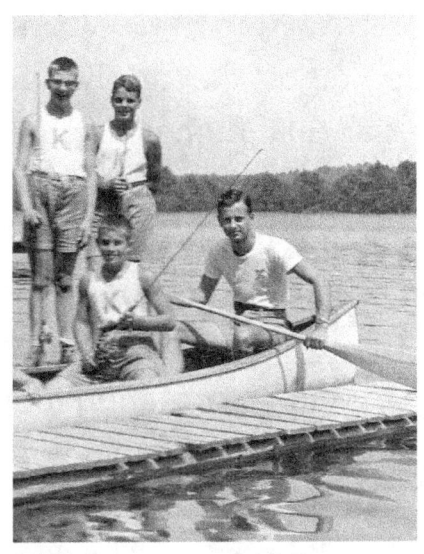

HEALTHY LIFESTYLE TIPS

"If I had known how old I was going to be I'd have taken better care of myself."

~ Adolf Zukor, founder of Paramount Pictures, before his 100th birthday

Annual Flu Shots

The Centers for Disease Control and Prevention report that adults aged 65 and older are at a higher risk for developing flu-related complications, such as pneumonia, bronchitis, sinus infections and ear infections. The CDC's website (www.cdc.gov) provides the most up-to-date information for each coming flu season, but what you need to know is that the best way to prevent the flu is with a flu vaccine. The CDC recommends that everyone 6 months of age and older get a seasonal flu vaccine as soon as it becomes available in your community. If you suspect you have developed the flu, seek medical help as soon as possible. Antiviral drugs can be administered, but they work best when used early.

Here are some tips from the CDC to help slow the spread of germs that cause respiratory illness, like the flu:

- Cover your nose and mouth with a tissue when you cough or sneeze. This will block the spread of droplets from your mouth or nose that could contain germs.
- Wash your hands often with soap and water. If soap and water are not available, use an alcohol-based hand rub.
- Avoid touching your eyes, nose and mouth. Germs spread this way.
- Try to avoid close contact with sick people.
- If you get the flu, limit contact with others as much as possible to help prevent spreading illness. Stay home for at least 24 hours after the fever is gone except to seek medical care or for other necessities. Fever should be gone without the use of a fever-reducing medicine.

How to Spot Signs of a Stroke

(Source: the American Stroke Association)

- Sudden numbness or weakness of the face, arm or leg, especially on one side of the body.

- Sudden confusion, trouble speaking or understanding.

- Sudden trouble seeing in one or both eyes.

- Sudden trouble walking, dizziness, loss of balance or coordination.

- Sudden severe headache with no known cause.

If you suspect someone is having a stroke, act quickly. There's a drug that, if administered within three hours of the first symptoms, can reduce the damage caused by the most common type of stroke. **Dial 9-1-1 immediately**.

Oral Health

According to the CDC, nearly one-third of all adults in the United States have untreated tooth decay. One in every four adults aged 65 years and older has gum disease, and oral cancers are most common in older adults, particularly those over 55 years who smoke and are heavy drinkers. Many older Americans take medications for chronic conditions that have side effects detrimental to their oral health, for example, antihistamines, diuretics and antidepressants.

Tips to Maintain Good Oral Health

- Drink fluoridated water and use fluoride toothpaste; fluoride provides protection against dental decay at all ages.

- Careful tooth brushing and flossing to reduce dental plaque can help prevent periodontal disease.

- If you have dentures, remove and clean every night and after each meal to reduce the risk of yeast and fungal infections.

- See your dentist on a regular basis, even if you have no natural teeth and have dentures. Professional care helps to maintain the overall health of the teeth and mouth, and provides for early detection of pre-cancerous or cancerous lesions.

- Avoid tobacco in any form. In addition to the general health risks posed by tobacco use, smokers have seven times the risk of developing periodontal disease compared to non-smokers. In addition, spit tobacco containing sugar increases the risk of cavities.

- Limit alcohol. Drinking a high amount of alcoholic beverages is a risk factor for oral and throat cancers. Alcohol and tobacco used together are the primary risk factors for these cancers.

- If medications produce a dry mouth, ask your doctor if there are other drugs that can be substituted. If dry mouth cannot be avoided, drink plenty of water, chew sugarless gum, and avoid tobacco and alcohol.

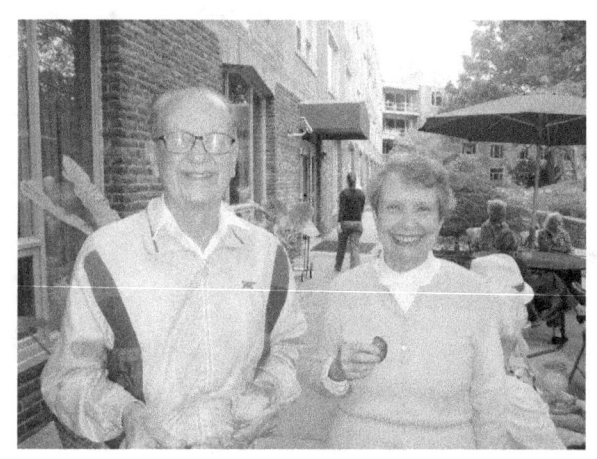

CONCLUSION

"True enjoyment comes from activity
of the mind and exercise of the body:
the two are ever united."

~ Karl Wilhelm von Humboldt

I was fortunate enough to have a family that encouraged exercise. My parents brought me and my siblings up on the tennis courts and gave us the benefit of appreciating a more active and participatory

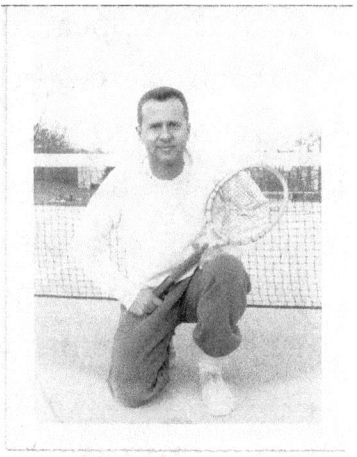

lifestyle at a young age – and that appreciation has remained with me as I've aged. Teaching your children your favorite exercise gives them a good start toward being more contributory members of society.

And I'm proof that the right kind of exercise and diet can stop you from aging prematurely. I see so many people aging too rapidly, looking much more than their chronological years. Increasing your activity will increase your youthful appearance. Have a regular exercise regimen to maximize your health and longevity. It's important to adhere to a program that's beneficial to you – smoking and excessive alcohol consumption is not helpful to your health and increase the aging process. So, make the decision to start a routine. Start slowly. Instead of doing nothing while you sit and watch TV, take that time to do some simple exercises. I spend about 40 minutes on the exercycle while watching TV and it helps me sleep better and get more benefit from my sleep. Overall, a regular routine can help you get more enjoyment out of life – throughout the week, my exercise routine includes pool therapy, pool aerobics, senior fitness classes and yoga. I feel in great shape and rejuvenated after exercise.

Sadly, one of my neighbors, who was just four years younger than me, passed away much earlier than I think he should have had he exercised regularly. He played a little golf but didn't do much more. Walking each day instead of riding a golf cart all the time is better advised.

Another neighbor fell and injured his leg. As a result, his daughter was caring for him and walking his dog. I believe, with regular aerobic (heart-lung benefit) exercise, his injury may not have been as severe. Especially with aerobic exercise, you are likely to suffer fewer injuries from falls because the muscles and bones are stronger. Keep in mind, of course, that bones get frail as we get older and we must take certain precautions that you don't think about when you are younger – for example, taking extra calcium to keep your bones strong. There's a gentleman who comes to the pool therapy class and he has been wearing dark glasses because he's getting his eyes treated. I was impressed to see him – he's a gutsy guy still getting in the pool and not letting the eye treatment stop him from being active.

Exercise lifts the spirits. As people feel better about themselves and feel the benefits of these activities, they become more contributory to society – people can contribute more than they realize once they get going. There are so many benefits to being a better contributor to society and raising the level of enthusiasm and interest of those around you. The elderly can have as much enthusiasm as younger people by simply being more engaged, socializing, being involved, and meeting people of different cultures and perspectives. There are endless possibilities out there, however, the average person doesn't look at life that way. They go to work and go home, but there's a lot more that can be done than they realize.

Maintain a social life! Too many spend their days in retirement homes just sitting around. Take advantage of the social opportunities available to you – bus trips, performances, theatre, or sports activities. Join a dance club or a swimming class – I'm always surprised at the few who come to our pool therapy classes, especially the lack of men who participate. Find friends with similar interests who will join you in a runners club, walking group, swim group, or tennis.

There are competitions to really invigorate people and get them on a more positive and healthful path, such as Senior Olympics.

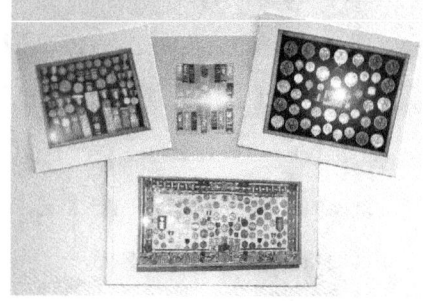

Don't wait for someone to come and talk to you. Go out and meet others. Don't just sit around, get out and do something! It can make all the difference to a longer, healthier life.

People should continue with
their education. Oftentimes, once
they get out of high school or
college, they are finished. The
higher education you have, the
better opportunities you have in
life. I've gone farther than the
average person because I took
advantage of opportunities that
came my way – I was fortunate to
receive six years of education using
the GI Bill. There are opportunities
all around – oftentimes classes are
available at your local hospital or
community college for free or at a
reduced senior citizen price – take
advantage of them. Don't forget to
share with others – if you help
someone, maybe that person will
help you. I mentored a young
woman while she was studying for
her doctorate and she, in turn,
recommended me for my doctoral

program.

There is much we can do to help ourselves and others live healthier lives. Find what works for you, and get out there and do it. And most of all, have fun!

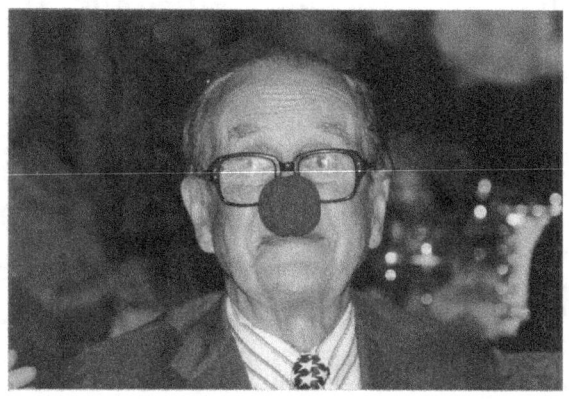

ABOUT THE AUTHOR

W. Newlin Hewson, Ph.D., is a retired senior military officer and civil servant. He entered the United States Air Force and served in World War II. He later worked with the U.S. Department of Housing and Urban Develop-ment and earned his Ph.D. for "The Prediction of FHA Home Mortgage Foreclosures," from Walden University in 1973.

He has been an active member of the American Statistical Association, the Operations Research Society of America, the American Association for the Advancement of Science, and Toastmasters International (President Emeritus of the Department of HUD Chapter).

Dr. Hewson has dedicated his life to enhancing the health and physical fitness of himself and others, and served as a health and fitness lecturer from 1982 to 1996. He currently resides in the Knollwood Military Officers Retirement Residence in Washington, D.C. And with the first edition, he became the first to publish a book while at Knollwood.